Mastering the Art of Foot care Nursing

By

Chad Peterson

Copyright © 2013

Introduction

Welcome to "Mastering the Art of Foot care Nursing," a comprehensive guide designed to empower nurses, healthcare professionals, and students with the knowledge and skills needed to excel in the specialized field of foot care. With the increasing demand for specialized foot care services, especially among populations such as the elderly and those with diabetes, the importance of skilled foot care nurses has never been greater.

This book is the culmination of years of experience and learning in the field of foot care nursing, combined with a deep commitment to patient care and education. As a Registered Practical Nurse and certified Advanced Foot Care Nurse, I have witnessed firsthand the profound impact that expert foot care can have on a patient's quality of life. It is this experience that I bring to these pages, aiming to equip you with both the technical skills and the compassionate approach required in this profession.

"Mastering the Art of Foot care Nursing" covers a wide range of topics essential for effective practice. From the basics of anatomy and common foot conditions to advanced techniques in managing complex cases, the content is structured to provide a step-by-step guide to everything you need to know. Additionally, this book addresses the often-overlooked aspects of foot care nursing, such as building patient relationships, ethical considerations, and the importance of continuing education in this evolving field.

Whether you are a nursing student eager to explore a potential specialty, a seasoned nurse looking to expand your skills, or a healthcare provider involved in patient care, this book offers valuable insights and practical advice to enhance your competence and confidence in providing foot care. Through clear explanations, case studies, and detailed illustrations, you will gain the tools to make a significant difference in the lives of your patients.

Join me in exploring the art and science of foot care nursing. Together, we will delve into the techniques, challenges, and rewards of a field that, while often understated, is essential to patient health and mobility. Let's step forward into mastering the skills that will elevate your practice and transform your patients' lives.

- **Foot Fun Facts:** Learn that each foot's complex structure includes 26 bones, 33 joints, and over 100 muscles, tendons, and ligaments, making up nearly a quarter of all the bones in the human body. Discover the astounding fact that feet can produce up to a pint of sweat each day and explore why such robust features are critical in nursing care.

- **Nursing Focus:** Tailored specifically for nurses, this guide covers the essentials of foot care nursing, from routine checks to managing diabetes-related foot complications. It underscores the importance of feet in assessing overall health and how foot health can reflect the state of the body.

- **Practical Care Strategies:** Equip yourself with practical knowledge and skills on preventative care, treatment of common foot ailments, and specialized techniques for managing chronic conditions. Learn how to conduct thorough assessments, choose appropriate interventions, and educate patients on maintaining foot health.

1. "The human foot is a masterpiece of engineering and a work of art."

- **Leonardo da Vinci** This quote celebrates the intricate and beautiful design of the human foot, admired by one of the greatest artists and thinkers of the Renaissance.

2. **"When your feet hurt, you hurt all over."**

- **Socrates** This quote from the ancient philosopher emphasizes the importance of foot health, highlighting how pain in your feet can affect your overall well-being.

3. **"Walking is man's best medicine."**

    - **Hippocrates** Here, the father of medicine, Hippocrates, reminds us of the fundamental role that walking, and by extension our feet, plays in maintaining health.

4. **"Our feet are our body's connection to the earth."**

    - **Andrew Weil** This quote from the American doctor reflects on the fundamental connection between our physical presence and the earth, mediated through our feet.

5. **"I cried because I had no shoes, then I met a man who had no feet."**

    - **Persian Proverb** This proverb offers a poignant perspective on gratitude and the relative nature of personal struggles.

6. **"The foot feels the foot when it feels the ground."**

    - **Buddha** Buddha's words here are a meditation on awareness and presence, noting how our feet connect us physically and sensibly to the world.

7. **"Stand on your own feet, and stand tall."**

    - **Unknown** This motivational quote encourages self-reliance and confidence, metaphorically using the act of standing as a symbol for personal strength.

1. **Introduction to Footcare Nursing**
    - Overview of the field
    - The importance of foot health in overall well-being
    - Scope of practice and ethical considerations

2. **Anatomy of the Foot**
    - Detailed review of foot anatomy including bones, muscles, joints, nerves, and circulation
    - Common anatomical variations and their clinical significance

3. **Assessment Techniques in Footcare**
    - Physical examination steps
    - Diagnostic tools and their applications
    - Patient history taking and its importance

4. **Common Foot Conditions**
    - Identification and management of disorders like diabetic foot, plantar fasciitis, bunions, and fungal infections
    - Case studies for practical understanding

5. **Wound Care Management**
    - Techniques for managing various types of foot wounds

- Dressing choices, infection control, and monitoring healing

6. **Footcare for Special Populations**
    - Tailoring care approaches for diabetics, elderly patients, and those with arterial or venous diseases
    - Preventive strategies to avoid complications

7. **Orthotics and Prosthetics**
    - Understanding the use and benefits of orthotics and prosthetic devices in footcare
    - Fitting, adjusting, and patient education

8. **Pharmacological Treatments**
    - Common medications used in footcare and their indications
    - Managing side effects and ensuring patient compliance

9. **Surgical Interventions**
    - Overview of surgical options for chronic and acute foot problems
    - Pre-operative and post-operative care

10. **Preventive Care and Patient Education**
    - Strategies to educate patients on maintaining foot health
    - Developing comprehensive care plans

11. Advancements in Footcare Nursing

- o Latest research, technologies, and trends in footcare
- o Future directions in therapy and patient management

12. Building a Footcare Practice

- o Essentials of setting up and managing a successful footcare practice
- o Legal, business, and marketing considerations for growth

13. Ethics and Professionalism in Footcare Nursing

- o Discussing ethical dilemmas specific to footcare
- o Maintaining professionalism and empathy in clinical practice

14. Conclusion: The Future of Footcare Nursing

- o Reflecting on the evolving role of footcare nurses
- o Encouraging continuous education and specialization

Dedication

This book is dedicated to the tireless nurses who continually seek to expand their scope of practice, acquire new skills, and create opportunities for self-employment within the ever-evolving field of healthcare. Your dedication to learning and growth is a beacon of inspiration.

To all the diabetic and elderly populations who suffer from neglected foot care—this book aims to shine a light on the importance of foot health and provide the care you need and deserve. It is for those who face daily challenges with courage and resilience, and for whom we strive to prevent future foot problems.

May this guide serve as a resource to empower nurses and patients alike, fostering enhanced care practices and promoting better health outcomes. Here's to mastering the art of foot care nursing, reducing the burden of foot ailments, and improving quality of life for susceptible demographics across the globe.

Ode to the Feet

Beneath the weight of bodies tall, Quietly, our feet bear all. They tread the earth with silent grace, Marking time and holding place.

Foundation firm on rocky trails, Over mountains, through the dales, Softly stepping on the sand, Guiding us with gentle hand.

They dance in joy, they shuffle in blues, In tired evenings, in worn-out shoes, They feel the pulse of pebbled streets, The chill of frost, the summer's heats.

Oh, faithful stewards of our strides, Through bustling days and peaceful tides, In every leap and every stance, You weave the steps of life's grand dance.

From tender toes of newborn's rest, To aged arches, doing their best, Every journey, every roam, Starts and ends with you, at home.

So here's to you, who do not sleep, A steadfast vigil, you always keep, Oh wondrous feet, with you, we fly, Till our final rest, when we say goodbye.

By Chad Peterson

Chapter 1: Introduction to Foot care Nursing

Learning Objectives

1. Understand the scope and significance of foot care nursing within the broader field of healthcare.

2. Recognize the impact of foot health on overall well-being and quality of life.

3. Identify the ethical considerations and scope of practice for foot care nurses.

Overview of Foot care Nursing

Foot care nursing is a specialized area within nursing that focuses on the assessment, care, and treatment of foot health issues. This field plays a crucial role in preventive health care, particularly for populations such as the elderly, diabetics, and those with chronic illnesses, where mobility and quality of life are significantly impacted by foot health.

The Importance of Foot Health in Overall Well-Being

The health of one's feet has a profound impact on overall well-being. As the foundation of mobility, healthy feet enable independence, facilitate physical activity, and significantly influence one's ability to participate in daily activities. Poor foot health can lead to pain, impairment, and reduced quality of life. For example, common conditions like bunions, corns, and toenail issues, while often considered minor, can lead to significant discomfort and mobility problems.

Scope of Practice and Ethical Considerations

Foot care nursing involves various responsibilities from routine checks and basic care (like trimming nails and treating minor skin issues) to more complex care strategies involving wound care, infection control, and managing chronic conditions such as diabetic foot ulcers. The scope of practice for a foot care nurse is defined by local regulations and typically requires specific training and certification in foot care

Ethically, foot care nurses are bound to uphold the same standards as other nursing professionals, which include maintaining patient dignity, ensuring informed consent, and providing care that is in the best interest of the patient. They must also navigate the complexities of treating patients who may have reduced sensation in their feet, such as those with diabetes, making communication and patient education crucial.

Summary of Lessons Learned

This chapter introduced the specialized field of foot care nursing, highlighting its importance in maintaining and improving patient mobility and overall health. Key lessons include:

- The critical role of foot health in overall physical well-being.

- The diverse scope of practice within foot care nursing, requiring specialized knowledge and skills.

- The ethical obligations that foot care nurses hold to ensure patient-centered and respectful care.

Understanding these foundational elements sets the stage for more detailed exploration of specific foot conditions, treatment strategies, and the nurse's role in patient education and preventive care in subsequent chapters.

References

1. American Association of Colleges of Nursing. (n.d.). Scope of practice.

2. National Institute on Aging. (2020). Foot care.

3. Nursing Ethics. (2019). Ethical considerations in nursing practice.

This chapter framework ensures a thorough introduction to the profession of foot care nursing, laying the groundwork for a deeper dive into specific practices and techniques used within this nursing specialty.

Chapter 2: Anatomy of the Foot

Learning Objectives

1. Gain a comprehensive understanding of the structural anatomy of the foot, including its bones, muscles, joints, nerves, and vascular supply.

2. Identify common anatomical variations in the foot and understand their clinical relevance and implications for foot care

3. Enhance diagnostic skills by correlating foot anatomy with common foot ailments and conditions.

Detailed Review of Foot Anatomy

Bones of the Foot

The foot consists of 26 bones, divided into three categories:

- **Tarsal bones**: Seven bones including the calcaneus (heel bone), talus, navicular, cuboid, and three cuneiform bones, forming the ankle and rear foot.

- **Metatarsal bones**: Five bones forming the middle part of the foot.

- **Phalanges**: Fourteen bones in the toes, with three in each toe except for the big toe, which has two.

Muscles of the Foot

Foot muscles are categorized into intrinsic and extrinsic groups:

- **Intrinsic muscles** originate and insert within the foot and are crucial for fine motor actions like toe movements.

- **Extrinsic muscles** originate in the lower leg and insert into various parts of the foot, controlling movements such as flexion and extension of the foot and toes.

Joints and Ligaments

The foot contains numerous joints, including the ankle joint (tibiotalar joint), subtalar joint, intertarsal joints, metatarsophalangeal joints, and interphalangeal joints. These joints are supported by a complex network of ligaments that maintain stability and facilitate movement.

Nerves and Circulation

- **Nerves**: Major nerves include the posterior tibial nerve, dorsalis pedis nerve, and the deep peroneal nerve, which innervate different parts of the foot and are responsible for sensory and motor functions.

- **Vascular supply**: The foot's blood supply comes primarily from the posterior tibial artery and the dorsalis pedis artery, ensuring adequate blood flow necessary for tissue health and healing.

Common Anatomical Variations and Their Clinical Significance

Some common variations include a high arch (pes cavus), flat feet (pes planus), and the presence of accessory bones such as the os trigonum. These variations can influence the risk of certain conditions, such as:

- **High arches** being associated with metatarsalgia and plantar fasciitis.

- **Flat feet** potentially leading to heel pain, arch strain, or overpronation-related injuries.

Summary of Lessons Learned

In this chapter, we have thoroughly explored the complex anatomy of the foot, which is foundational for understanding how to assess, diagnose, and treat foot conditions effectively. Key lessons include:

- The structural intricacy of foot anatomy, involving bones, muscles, joints, nerves, and blood vessels.

- The clinical importance of recognizing anatomical variations and their potential impact on foot health and susceptibility to specific foot disorders.

References

- Gray's Anatomy for Students, 3rd Edition. Elsevier Health Sciences.

- Clinically Oriented Anatomy, Keith L. Moore, et al.

- Podiatry Institute, Foot and Ankle Anatomy.

This chapter offers an essential foundation for any foot care professional, providing the anatomical knowledge necessary to understand common foot issues and perform effective interventions.

Chapter 3: Assessment Techniques in Foot care Nursing

Learning Objectives

1. Master the steps involved in conducting a comprehensive physical examination of the foot.

2. Understand the use and significance of various diagnostic tools in foot care

3. Appreciate the importance of thorough patient history taking and its impact on foot care outcomes.

Physical Examination Steps

The physical examination of the foot is a systematic process that involves several key steps:

- **Visual Inspection**: Assess the overall appearance of the foot for any abnormalities such as swelling, discoloration, or structural deformities.

- **Palpation**: Feel the foot to detect any abnormalities in the bones, joints, and soft tissues. This helps in identifying areas of tenderness or pain.

- **Range of Motion Tests**: Evaluate the mobility of the joints in the foot and ankle to check for stiffness, pain, or other limitations.

- **Neurological Examination**: Check for sensory and motor function to assess nerve health, especially important in patients with diabetes.

- **Vascular Assessment**: Examine the pulses in the foot to ensure good blood flow. This includes palpating the dorsalis pedis and the posterior tibial arteries.

Diagnostic Tools and Their Applications

Several diagnostic tools are essential in the assessment of foot health:

- **Gait Analysis**: Observing the patient's walking pattern can help identify abnormalities and guide corrective measures.

- **X-rays**: Essential for visualizing bone structure and identifying fractures, deformities, or signs of arthritis.

- **Ultrasound**: Used for assessing soft tissue structures and diagnosing issues such as tendon tears or soft tissue masses.

- **MRI**: Offers detailed images of both hard and soft tissues, providing comprehensive information about complex foot conditions.

Importance of Patient History Taking

Taking a comprehensive patient history is crucial and includes:

- **Medical History**: Information about systemic health conditions, such as diabetes or rheumatoid arthritis, which can affect foot health.

- **Medication Review**: Some medications can influence foot health, for example, steroids can weaken tissues.

- **Lifestyle and Activity Level**: Insights into the patient's daily activities and occupational demands can guide treatment planning.

- **History of Present Illness**: Detailed descriptions of the current foot problems, including the onset, duration, and severity of symptoms.

Summary of Lessons Learned

This chapter emphasized the critical role of proper assessment techniques in foot care nursing. Key takeaways include:

- The systematic approach to physical examinations ensures no aspect of foot health is overlooked.

- Diagnostic tools, when used appropriately, enhance the understanding and treatment of foot conditions.

- Comprehensive patient history is indispensable, providing context and aiding in accurate diagnosis and effective management.

References

- "Clinical Examination of the Foot and Ankle" by Dr. Paul D. Smith - This book provides insights into detailed examination techniques.

- "Podiatric Assessment and Diagnosis" by Marianne T. L. Smith - Offers guidelines on the use of various diagnostic tools.

- Journal of Foot and Ankle Research - Contains numerous articles on the latest diagnostic technologies and their applications in foot care

Understanding and applying these assessment techniques effectively sets the foundation for successful treatment outcomes in foot care nursing, ensuring that care is both appropriate and holistic.

Chapter 4: Identification and Management of Common Foot Disorders

Diabetic Foot

- **Identification**: Characterized by poor circulation, loss of sensation, foot ulcers, and infections.

- **Management**: Regular monitoring for sores or changes in foot appearance, maintaining good foot hygiene, controlling blood sugar levels, and using diabetic-specific footwear.

  - *Nursing Interventions for Diabetic Foot Care*

1. **Regular Inspection and Monitoring:**

   o Perform daily inspections of the patient's feet for any signs of injury, infection, or changes such as cuts, blisters, redness, or swelling.

   o Use a mirror or assist in checking areas of the feet that are hard to see.

2. **Management of Blood Glucose:**

   o Monitor blood glucose levels as part of the routine care plan.

   o Collaborate with the healthcare team to adjust medications or dietary plans to maintain optimal blood glucose control.

3. **Wound Care:**

- Cleanse wounds using sterile techniques to prevent infection.
- Apply appropriate dressings to promote healing and prevent further damage.
- Ensure timely referral to a wound care specialist when needed.

4. **Infection Control:**
    - Administer antibiotics as prescribed if signs of infection are present.
    - Educate the patient on the signs of infection to watch for and when to seek immediate care.

5. **Skin and Nail Care:**
    - Trim nails carefully or advise a podiatrist visit if nails are thickened or difficult to cut.
    - Apply moisturizers to dry skin but avoid lotion between the toes to reduce infection risk.

Nursing Considerations for Diabetic Foot Care

1. **Assessment Skills:**
    - Be vigilant in assessing the neurological and vascular status of the feet. Neuropathy can often mask injuries due to reduced sensation.
    - Conduct regular foot exams and utilize tools like monofilaments to test sensitivity.

2. **Individualized Care Planning:**

- Recognize that each patient's needs may differ depending on their level of mobility, risk of ulceration, and history of foot problems.
- Adjust care plans based on individual risk assessments and patient feedback.

3. **Coordination of Care:**

    - Coordinate with a multidisciplinary team including podiatrists, endocrinologists, and dietitians to provide comprehensive care.
    - Arrange for appropriate footwear advice or orthotics if required.

Client Education for Diabetic Foot Care

1. **Daily Foot Care Routine:**

    - Instruct patients on how to inspect their feet daily using mirrors to check all areas.
    - Teach proper foot washing techniques, using lukewarm water and drying thoroughly, especially between the toes.

2. **Importance of Footwear:**

    - Advise on the selection of well-fitting, comfortable shoes and the avoidance of walking barefoot.
    - Recommend wearing clean, dry socks without tight elastic bands.

3. **Lifestyle Modifications:**

- - Discuss the importance of smoking cessation as smoking worsens peripheral vascular disease.
  - Encourage regular, gentle exercise to improve blood circulation.

4. **Emergency Education:**

    - Educate patients on recognizing the signs of infection or severe ulcers and the importance of prompt treatment.
    - Provide clear instructions on when and how to seek help in an emergency.

By implementing these nursing interventions, considering individual patient needs, and educating clients effectively, healthcare providers can significantly reduce the risks associated with diabetic foot complications and promote better overall foot health in diabetic patients.

-

Plantar Fasciitis

- **Identification**: Presents with sharp heel pain, typically worse in the morning.
- **Management**: Stretching exercises, proper footwear, orthotics, anti-inflammatory medications, and in persistent cases, corticosteroid injections.

    - *Nursing Interventions for Plantar Fasciitis*

1. **Pain Management:**

- Administer pain relief medications as prescribed, such as NSAIDs (Nonsteroidal Anti-Inflammatory Drugs) to reduce inflammation and pain.
- Recommend cold therapy, such as applying ice packs to the affected area for 15-20 minutes several times a day to reduce swelling.

2. **Physical Support:**
    - Assist in the fitting and use of supportive devices like orthotics or heel pads that help distribute pressure away from the plantar fascia.
    - Encourage the use of supportive footwear that has good arch support and cushioning.

3. **Referral for Physical Therapy:**
    - Coordinate referrals to physical therapy for targeted exercises aimed at stretching the plantar fascia and Achilles tendon, and strengthening lower leg muscles, which stabilize the ankle and heel.

Nursing Considerations for Plantar Fasciitis

1. **Individual Assessment:**
    - Evaluate the patient's foot structure, type of daily activities, and any underlying health conditions that may contribute to the condition, such as obesity or occupations requiring long hours on the feet.
    - Assess pain levels regularly to monitor progress and effectiveness of interventions.

2. **Lifestyle and Occupational Factors:**

- Consider the patient's lifestyle and occupational needs when recommending modifications or supportive devices.
- Work with the patient to adjust routines that may exacerbate the condition, such as standing for long periods or engaging in high-impact activities.

3. **Monitoring for Complications:**

    - Keep an eye on signs of complications, such as increased pain, changes in walking patterns, or signs of depression due to chronic pain, and coordinate care accordingly.

Client Education for Plantar Fasciitis

1. **Exercise and Stretching:**

    - Educate patients on specific exercises that can relieve plantar fasciitis pain, such as toe stretches, calf stretches, and towel stretches.
    - Advise on the importance of regular gentle exercise to improve blood flow, which aids in tissue healing.

2. **Proper Footwear:**

    - Instruct patients on choosing shoes with adequate support and padding. Advise avoiding flat shoes and walking barefoot on hard surfaces.
    - Discuss the potential need for custom orthotics, particularly for patients with severe symptoms or those not responding to over-the-counter options.

3. **Weight Management:**

- Discuss the impact of weight on foot health. Encourage strategies for weight loss if obesity is a contributing factor, as this can significantly decrease stress on the plantar fascia.

4. **Activity Modification:**
    - Teach patients about the importance of balancing rest and activity. Advise them to avoid activities that cause pain, such as prolonged standing or running.
    - Encourage the incorporation of low-impact activities like swimming or cycling, which do not put excessive stress on the feet.

5. **Pain Management Techniques:**
    - Educate on the use of ice packs for inflammation and techniques for proper application to avoid skin damage.
    - Discuss the appropriate use of over-the-counter pain medications, focusing on dosing and the potential side effects.

By integrating these nursing interventions, considerations, and educational strategies, healthcare providers can help patients manage plantar fasciitis effectively, reducing pain and improving their overall quality of life.

-

Bunions

- **Identification**: Bony bump on the joint at the base of the big toe, causing toe misalignment.

- **Management**: Wearing wider shoes with adequate toe room, orthotics, pain relievers, and surgery in severe cases.

  - *Nursing Interventions for Bunions*

1. **Pain Management:**

   o Administer or recommend pain relief medications as prescribed, such as NSAIDs (Nonsteroidal Anti-Inflammatory Drugs) to help manage inflammation and discomfort.

   o Apply or suggest cold packs to the affected area to reduce swelling and alleviate pain.

2. **Physical Support:**

   o Assist in the fitting and use of orthotic devices or bunion pads that can help redistribute pressure away from the bunion and alleviate discomfort.

   o Encourage the use of comfortable, well-fitting footwear with a wide toe box that minimizes pressure on the bunion.

3. **Referral for Physical Therapy or Surgery:**

   o Coordinate referrals to physical therapy for exercises that can maintain joint mobility and prevent stiffness or worsening of the bunion.

   o Discuss and prepare the patient for potential surgical interventions if conservative treatments are ineffective, especially in severe cases.

Nursing Considerations for Bunions

1. **Individual Assessment:**

    o   Evaluate the patient's foot structure and gait to understand contributing factors such as pronation or flat feet, which may exacerbate the bunion.

    o   Regularly assess pain and mobility levels to monitor progression and effectiveness of interventions.

2. **Lifestyle and Occupational Factors:**

    o   Consider the patient's daily activities and occupational demands when recommending modifications or supportive devices.

    o   Work with the patient to adjust routines that may exacerbate the condition, such as minimizing time spent in high heels or constrictive shoes.

3. **Monitoring for Complications:**

    o   Monitor for signs of complications such as increased pain, changes in toe alignment, or the development of secondary issues like bursitis or hammertoe.

Client Education for Bunions

1. **Exercise and Stretching:**

    o   Educate patients on specific exercises that can help maintain joint mobility and alleviate discomfort, such as toe stretches and range-of-motion exercises.

    o   Advise on the importance of avoiding exercises that put excessive pressure on the feet.

2. **Proper Footwear:**

- o Instruct patients on selecting appropriate footwear that offers good support and a wide toe box to accommodate the bunion and reduce pressure.
- o Discuss the benefits of custom orthotics for providing additional support and alleviating pressure on the bunion.

3. **Activity Modification:**

   - o Teach patients about the importance of balancing rest and activity to manage pain and prevent worsening of the bunion.
   - o Encourage the patient to choose low-impact activities that do not exacerbate the condition.

4. **Pain Management Techniques:**

   - o Educate on the use of ice packs for managing inflammation and techniques for proper application.
   - o Discuss the appropriate use of over-the-counter pain medications, focusing on dosing and potential side effects.

By integrating these nursing interventions, considerations, and educational strategies, healthcare providers can help patients manage bunions effectively, aiming to reduce discomfort, prevent progression, and improve overall foot health and mobility.

-

Seed Corns

- **Identification**: Small, concentrated areas of hard skin, typically found on drier parts of the foot like the heel.

- **Management**: Salicylic acid treatments, wearing cushioned pads, and in some cases, minor surgery to remove the corn.

Nursing Interventions for Seed Corns

1. **Pain Management:**

   o Administer or recommend over-the-counter pain relief medications, such as acetaminophen or NSAIDs (Nonsteroidal Anti-Inflammatory Drugs), to help manage discomfort.

   o Advise the use of cushioned pads or moleskin around the corn to relieve pressure and reduce pain.

2. **Physical Support:**

   o Assist in the selection and fitting of orthotic devices that can help redistribute pressure away from the corn.

   o Encourage the use of well-fitting, comfortable footwear that does not compress the feet, focusing on shoes with a wide toe box.

3. **Careful Trimming:**

   o If appropriate and within the scope of practice, gently pare down the corn with a sterile scalpel, but only after soaking and softening the area. This should be done cautiously and preferably by a healthcare professional to avoid damaging healthy surrounding skin.

Nursing Considerations for Seed Corns

1. **Individual Assessment:**

- o Evaluate the patient's foot structure, skin condition, and gait to identify factors contributing to corn formation, such as improper footwear or abnormal foot mechanics.

- o Regularly assess the condition of the corn, including any signs of infection or significant changes in appearance.

2. **Lifestyle and Occupational Factors:**

    - o Consider the patient's daily activities and occupational demands that may affect foot health. Adjustments in footwear or activity levels may be necessary to alleviate pressure on the affected area.

3. **Monitoring for Complications:**

    - o Keep an eye on signs of infection such as increased redness, pain, swelling, or pus, which would necessitate prompt medical attention.

Client Education for Seed Corns

1. **Proper Foot Care:**

    - o Educate patients on the importance of maintaining good foot hygiene and moisturizing to keep skin from becoming too dry and prone to corns.

    - o Instruct on the proper technique for safely soaking and softening corns at home, which can ease discomfort and facilitate healing.

2. **Appropriate Footwear:**

- Advise on selecting shoes that fit well and provide adequate support and cushioning. Discuss the detrimental effects of tight or high-heeled shoes on foot health.

3. **Self-Care Techniques:**
    - Teach patients how to safely use over-the-counter pads or cushions specifically designed for corns to protect the area and reduce pressure.
    - Discuss the importance of not attempting to cut or remove corns at home to prevent injuries and infections.

4. **When to Seek Further Help:**
    - Educate patients on recognizing signs that require professional intervention, such as persistent pain, signs of infection, or corns that do not improve with self-care measures.

By incorporating these nursing interventions, considerations, and educational strategies, healthcare providers can effectively support patients in managing seed corns, aiming to alleviate discomfort, prevent complications, and promote better foot health.

Hammer Toes and Claw Toes

- **Identification**: Toes bent into an abnormal position, often painful.

- **Management**: Corrective footwear, orthotics, toe pads or caps, and surgery for correction if causing significant pain or mobility issues.

Nursing Interventions for Hammer Toes and Claw Toes

1. **Pain Management:**

    - Administer or suggest over-the-counter pain relievers such as acetaminophen or NSAIDs (Nonsteroidal Anti-Inflammatory Drugs) to help manage discomfort.

    - Recommend the use of non-medicated padding to relieve pressure and reduce pain on the affected toes.

2. **Physical Support:**

    - Assist in the fitting of appropriate orthotic devices that can help correct the misalignment and distribute pressure evenly.

    - Encourage the use of proper footwear that provides adequate room for the toes, including shoes with a high and wide toe box to prevent further constriction.

3. **Referral for Physical Therapy:**

    - Coordinate referrals to physical therapy for targeted exercises designed to stretch and strengthen the muscles in the foot, which can help improve toe alignment and mobility.

Nursing Considerations for Hammer Toes and Claw Toes

1. **Individual Assessment:**
   - Evaluate the patient's foot anatomy, the severity of the toe deformity, and any contributing factors such as underlying neuromuscular diseases or previous injuries.
   - Regularly assess for changes in skin integrity, signs of calluses or ulcers, particularly in diabetic patients, due to altered foot mechanics.

2. **Lifestyle and Occupational Factors:**
   - Consider how the patient's daily activities and occupational demands may exacerbate their condition, advising on modifications to reduce strain on the toes.

3. **Monitoring for Complications:**
   - Monitor for complications such as worsening pain, increases in deformity, and signs of infection or significant callus formation that might require more aggressive interventions, possibly even surgical referral.

Client Education for Hammer Toes and Claw Toes

1. **Proper Footwear:**
   - Instruct patients on choosing footwear that fits properly and supports the foot without compressing the toes. Shoes should have a wide toe box that does not force the toes into a bent position.
   - Discuss the importance of avoiding high heels and tight shoes which can exacerbate the condition.

2. **Exercise and Foot Care:**
   - Teach specific exercises that can help stretch and strengthen the toes, such as towel curls and marble pickups.
   - Educate on the importance of foot care, including checking for and managing calluses and avoiding any self-treatment with over-the-counter remedies that might damage the skin, such as medicated corn pads.

3. **Use of Devices:**
   - Demonstrate how to correctly use toe spacers, bunion pads, or splints designed to keep toes in a more natural position and relieve pressure.
   - Advise on the temporary use of taping as a means to maintain correct toe alignment.

4. **When to Consider Surgery:**
   - Educate patients about the potential need for surgical interventions if conservative measures fail to relieve pain or if toe deformity becomes severe. Discuss what the surgical options involve and the typical outcomes.

By implementing these nursing interventions, considerations, and educational strategies, healthcare providers can effectively support patients with hammer toes and claw toes, aiming to relieve discomfort, prevent progression of deformities, and improve overall foot function and health.

Plantar Warts

- **Identification**: Hard, grainy growths on the soles of the feet, caused by the human papillomavirus (HPV).
- **Management**: Over-the-counter treatments, cryotherapy, or surgical removal.

Fungal Infections (Athlete's Foot)

- **Identification**: Itchy, red, cracked, and flaking skin, particularly between the toes.
- **Management**: Antifungal creams or pills, keeping feet dry and clean, and using antifungal powders in shoes.

Case Studies for Practical Understanding

- **Case Study 1**: A 58-year-old diabetic male with recurrent foot ulcers treated through improved glycemic control and protective footwear.
- **Case Study 2**: A 35-year-old runner diagnosed with plantar fasciitis, managed with physical therapy and custom orthotics.
- **Case Study 3**: A young adult with severe plantar warts treated with cryotherapy followed by salicylic acid applications.

Expanded Case Studies with Reflection Questions

Case Study 1: Managing Recurrent Foot Ulcers in a Diabetic Patient

Background: A 58-year-old male with a long-standing history of type 2 diabetes presents with recurrent foot ulcers. The patient has struggled with glycemic control, which has contributed to his chronic wound issues.

Intervention: The healthcare team focused on intensive glycemic control through medication adjustments, dietary consultations, and regular monitoring of blood glucose levels. Concurrently, the patient was fitted with therapeutic diabetic shoes and custom orthotic inserts to reduce pressure on susceptible areas of the feet.

Outcome: These interventions led to a significant improvement in the patient's blood sugar levels and a reduction in the recurrence of foot ulcers. The protective footwear helped prevent new ulcers by distributing weight more evenly and protecting sensitive areas from trauma.

Reflection Questions:

1. How might the patient's initial approach to managing his diabetes have contributed to the development of foot ulcers?

2. What role do you think patient education played in improving the patient's adherence to the new treatment plan?

3. How could the healthcare team further support the patient to prevent future complications?

Case Study 2: Plantar Fasciitis Management in a Runner

Background: A 35-year-old avid runner is diagnosed with plantar fasciitis after experiencing persistent heel pain. The condition threatens to keep her from participating in upcoming races.

Intervention: A treatment plan was developed that included physical therapy focusing on stretching exercises for the Achilles tendon and plantar fascia. The patient was also provided with custom orthotic inserts designed to correct foot alignment and distribute pressure more evenly during running.

Outcome: The combination of physical therapy and orthotics significantly alleviated the patient's pain, allowing her to gradually return to running. She reported improved comfort and reduced symptoms during her runs.

Reflection Questions:

1. Consider the psychological impact of plantar fasciitis on an avid runner. How might this affect her compliance with the treatment regimen?

2. Discuss the importance of foot biomechanics in the prevention and management of plantar fasciitis in athletes.

3. What preventive measures could the runner take to minimize the risk of recurrence?

Case Study 3: Treatment of Severe Plantar Warts

Background: A young adult patient presents with several painful and severe plantar warts that have not responded to over-the-counter treatments.

Intervention: The treatment strategy included an initial session of cryotherapy to freeze and kill the wart tissue, followed by the application of salicylic acid patches to further reduce the wart size. The patient was instructed on the correct application of the patches and the importance of regular skin care.

Outcome: After several treatment cycles, the warts significantly decreased in size and number, leading to pain relief and improved foot comfort.

Reflection Questions:

1. Why might home remedies or over-the-counter treatments fail in severe cases of plantar warts?

2. What are the potential risks of untreated plantar warts in young, active individuals?

3. How can patients be educated to prevent the spread of plantar warts within communal environments like gyms or pools?

These case studies with accompanying reflection questions are designed to deepen understanding of each condition and the effectiveness of various treatment approaches, while also encouraging critical thinking about broader implications and preventive strategies.

Summary of Lessons Learned

This chapter provided a thorough understanding of how to diagnose and manage common foot conditions effectively. It highlighted the importance of:

- Early identification and appropriate management to prevent complications.

- Tailoring treatment strategies to individual needs and conditions.

- Using case studies as a learning tool to see how theoretical knowledge is applied in practical settings.

References

- American Podiatric Medical Association. (n.d.). Podiatric conditions.

- National Institute of Diabetes and Digestive and Kidney Diseases. (n.d.). Diabetic neuropathy.

- Clinical guidelines on the identification, evaluation, and treatment of overweight and obesity in adults.

By mastering the content of this chapter, healthcare providers can enhance their competency in treating foot conditions, leading to improved patient outcomes and quality of life.

Chapter 5: Wound Care Management in Foot care Nursing

Learning Objectives

1. Understand the principles and techniques for managing various types of foot wounds.

2. Learn about different dressing options and their specific applications based on wound type and stage.

3. Master the strategies for infection control and effective monitoring of wound healing processes.

Techniques for Managing Various Types of Foot Wounds

Effective wound care management is crucial for preventing complications and promoting healing in foot wounds. The types of foot wounds commonly encountered in foot care nursing include diabetic ulcers, pressure ulcers, arterial and venous ulcers, and traumatic wounds.

- **Cleansing**: Proper wound cleansing is essential to remove contaminants and decrease the risk of infection. Use gentle cleansing solutions and techniques tailored to the wound type.

- **Debridement**: This involves the removal of dead or necrotic tissue, which is vital for promoting the growth of healthy new tissue. Methods include surgical, enzymatic, and autolytic debridement, depending on the wound condition.

- **Moisture Balance**: Maintaining the correct moisture balance with appropriate dressings aids in enhancing the wound healing environment.

Nursing Considerations for Wound Cleansing

1. **Assessment of Wound Characteristics:**

    - Evaluate the wound for size, depth, type of exudate, signs of infection, and surrounding skin condition. This will help determine the most appropriate cleansing solution and method.

    - Regularly assess the wound before and after cleansing to monitor for any changes or improvements.

2. **Selection of Cleansing Solutions:**

    - Choose a cleansing solution that is appropriate for the wound type. For most wounds, normal saline is preferred due to its safety and isotonic nature.

    - Avoid using cytotoxic agents like hydrogen peroxide or iodine-based solutions, which can damage granulation tissue, unless specifically indicated for certain infective conditions.

3. **Gentle Cleansing Techniques:**

    - Use gentle pressure to avoid trauma to the wound bed and surrounding tissues. Soft gauze or a bulb syringe can be effective for minimizing disruption to new tissue growth.

    - Ensure that the entire wound area and the surrounding skin are thoroughly cleansed to remove all contaminants and residues.

Nursing Considerations for Debridement

1. **Method Selection:**

    o Choose the debridement method based on the wound's condition, presence of necrotic tissue, and the patient's overall health status. For example, surgical debridement may be quick but requires professional expertise and can be painful, whereas autolytic debridement is gentler but slower.

    o Collaborate with wound care specialists when selecting a method, especially for complex wounds.

2. **Pain Management:**

    o Prioritize patient comfort and pain control before, during, and after debridement procedures. Administer pain relief medications as prescribed and monitor their effectiveness.

    o Prepare the patient psychologically by explaining the procedure and expected sensations.

3. **Monitoring for Complications:**

    o Regularly monitor the wound for signs of infection or increased exudate, which may indicate that the debridement method needs to be reassessed.

    o Keep detailed documentation of the wound's response to debridement to guide ongoing treatment decisions.

Nursing Considerations for Maintaining Moisture Balance

1. **Dressing Selection:**

- Select a dressing that appropriately manages the level of exudate while maintaining a moist wound environment. For example, use hydrocolloid dressings for wounds with minimal exudate and alginate or foam dressings for wounds with moderate to high exudate.
- Consider the wound stage, location, and patient's activity level when selecting a dressing to ensure it remains in place and functions effectively.

2. **Dressing Change Protocol:**

   - Develop and follow a standardized protocol for dressing changes that minimizes the risk of infection. Use aseptic techniques and change dressings as often as required based on the wound's exudate levels and the dressing manufacturer's instructions.
   - Educate the patient and caregivers on the correct procedure for dressing changes, especially if they are managing care at home.

3. **Hydration and Nutrition Support:**

   - Support overall skin and wound healing by encouraging adequate hydration and a balanced diet rich in protein, vitamins, and minerals essential for wound healing, such as Vitamin C, Zinc, and iron.
   - Consult with a nutritionist for patients with nutritional deficits to tailor dietary interventions that support wound healing.

By incorporating these nursing considerations into wound care practices, nurses can ensure comprehensive management that promotes healing, reduces complications, and enhances patient comfort and outcomes.

Dressing Choices

Choosing the right dressing is pivotal in managing any wound. The choice depends on the wound's exudate level, stage, and presence of infection.

- **Foam Dressings**: Ideal for wounds with moderate to high exudate, providing moisture retention and cushioning.

- **Hydrocolloid Dressings**: Used for wounds with mild to moderate exudate; these dressings promote moist wound healing and autolytic debridement.

- **Alginate Dressings**: Suitable for highly exudative wounds, these dressings absorb exudate and form a gel-like covering over the wound, maintaining a moist environment.

- **Antimicrobial Dressings**: Containing agents like silver or iodine, these are used when infection is present or at high risk.

Infection Control and Monitoring Healing

Infection control is a critical aspect of wound care, involving regular assessment, the use of sterile techniques during dressing changes, and appropriate antibiotic use when necessary.

- **Monitoring**: Regular assessment using tools like the PUSH (Pressure Ulcer Scale for Healing) tool to monitor changes in wound size, exudate, and tissue type.

- **Patient Education**: Teaching patients about signs of infection and the importance of proper foot hygiene can significantly impact recovery rates.

Summary of Lessons Learned

This chapter emphasized the importance of comprehensive wound care management, including proper assessment techniques, the judicious selection of wound dressings, and vigilant infection control measures. Key takeaways include:

- The importance of a tailored approach to wound management that considers the unique characteristics of each wound.

- The critical role of patient education and involvement in the wound care process.

- Continuous monitoring and adaptation of care plans based on wound healing progression.

References

- "Wound Care Essentials: Practice Principles" by Sharon Baranoski and Elizabeth A. Ayello.

- "Clinical Practice Guidelines for the Prediction and Prevention of Pressure Ulcers" by the National Pressure Ulcer Advisory Panel.

This chapter provides the foundational knowledge and practical skills necessary for effective wound management in foot care nursing, ensuring that professionals are equipped to handle complex wound care scenarios efficiently.

Chapter 6: Footrace for Special Populations

Learning Objectives

By the end of this chapter, readers will be able to:

1. Understand the specific foot care needs of diabetics, elderly patients, and individuals with arterial or venous diseases.

2. Identify common foot-related complications associated with these populations.

3. Apply tailored preventive strategies to minimize the risk of foot-related complications.

4. Recognize symptoms that require professional intervention.

Introduction

Footrace is essential for maintaining mobility and quality of life, particularly for populations with increased health risks. Diabetics, elderly individuals, and people with arterial or venous diseases face unique challenges that require specialized care to prevent complications. This chapter discusses tailored approaches to foot care for these groups and outlines effective preventive strategies.

Diabetic Footrace

Diabetes can cause nerve damage and reduced blood flow to the feet, making it difficult for injuries and infections to heal. Diabetic patients must adopt a rigorous foot care routine that includes:

Key Strategies:

- **Daily Inspections:** Checking feet daily for cuts, blisters, redness, or swelling.

- **Proper Footwear:** Wearing well-fitted shoes to avoid pressure sores.

- **Moisturizing and Hygiene:** Keeping feet clean and moisturized to prevent cracks.

- **Professional Check-ups:** Regular consultations with healthcare providers for professional foot examinations.

Nursing Interventions for Diabetic Foot Care

1. **Routine Monitoring and Assessment:**

    - Conduct regular and thorough inspections of the feet during each visit to check for any signs of cuts, blisters, redness, swelling, or infections.

    - Measure and document any changes in foot temperature, skin condition, and integrity to track progress or deterioration over time.

2. **Care Coordination:**

    - Schedule regular appointments with podiatrists for professional foot examinations. Ensure these visits are maintained as part of the ongoing diabetes management plan.

    - Coordinate with other healthcare providers, such as dietitians or diabetes educators, to provide a holistic approach to the patient's health.

3. **Wound Management:**

- Provide immediate care for any injuries found during inspections, using appropriate wound care techniques to prevent infection and promote healing.
- Educate patients on the importance of prompt treatment for foot injuries and the risks associated with delayed care.

Nursing Considerations for Diabetic Foot Care

1. **Risk Factor Management:**

   - Keep a close watch on patients with a history of ulcers or amputations, as they are at higher risk for complications. These patients may need more frequent monitoring.
   - Consider the patient's ability to bend and inspect their feet. Provide assistance or tools such as mirrors or foot inspection cameras if necessary.

2. **Patient Comfort and Compliance:**

   - Ensure that any footwear recommended is not only medically appropriate but also comfortable for the patient, as discomfort can lead to noncompliance.
   - Manage pain and discomfort associated with foot problems effectively to encourage patient adherence to recommended care practices.

3. **Lifestyle Modifications:**

   - Advise on lifestyle changes that can improve blood flow and overall diabetes control, such as regular exercise, smoking cessation, and maintaining a healthy weight.

Client Education for Diabetic Foot Care

1. **Daily Foot Care Routine:**

    - Instruct patients to wash their feet daily with lukewarm water and mild soap, drying thoroughly, especially between the toes.

    - Teach them to moisturize their feet to prevent dry skin and cracks but to avoid applying lotion between toes to reduce the risk of fungal infections.

2. **Proper Footwear:**

    - Educate patients on choosing shoes that fit well and provide adequate support without causing pressure points. Discuss the importance of avoiding walking barefoot to prevent injuries.

    - Recommend diabetic-specific footwear for those with significant deformities or history of ulcers.

3. **Self-Inspection Techniques:**

    - Demonstrate how to inspect feet properly using a mirror to check all areas. Emphasize looking for skin color changes, cuts, sores, or any signs of infection.

    - Educate patients on what signs to look for and when to seek immediate medical help.

4. **Professional Care and Follow-Up:**

    - Stress the importance of regular check-ups with healthcare providers to monitor the health of their feet.

- o Encourage patients to maintain their scheduled appointments and discuss any concerns they have about their feet or general health.

By integrating these interventions, considerations, and educational strategies, nurses can empower diabetic patients to take an active role in managing their foot health, thus preventing complications and promoting better overall outcomes.

Footrace for the Elderly

As individuals age, skin elasticity and cushioning around the feet decrease, increasing vulnerability to injuries. Elderly foot care should focus on:

Key Strategies:

- **Safe Footwear:** Shoes with non-slip soles and proper support.
- **Regular Exercise:** Activities that enhance blood circulation and foot strength.
- **Gentle Handling:** Avoiding injury during nail trimming and skin care.

Nursing Interventions for Elderly Foot Care

1. **Routine Monitoring and Assessment:**
   - o Conduct regular inspections of the elderly patients' feet to check for any signs of cuts, blisters, redness, swelling, or infections.

- Assess skin integrity, noting any changes in moisture (too dry or too moist), the presence of calluses, corns, and ulcers.

2. **Care Coordination:**

    - Facilitate regular consultations with podiatrists for professional foot examinations and coordinate care with physical therapists to enhance mobility and foot strength.

    - Ensure any signs of neuropathy or circulation issues are addressed by appropriate specialists.

3. **Injury Prevention:**

    - Provide guidance on safe practices for nail trimming and skin care to prevent injuries. Use gentle techniques and avoid aggressive cutting.

Nursing Considerations for Elderly Foot Care

1. **Footwear and Support:**

    - Assist in selecting footwear that provides stability, support, and non-slip soles to prevent falls. Ensure shoes fit well and accommodate any foot deformities without causing pressure points.

    - Consider the use of custom orthotic devices if standard footwear does not adequately address the patient's needs.

2. **Mobility and Safety:**

    - Encourage activities and exercises that are safe and effective for improving blood circulation and

strengthening the feet, considering the patient's overall mobility and balance capabilities.
- o Implement safety measures in the living environment to reduce the risk of falls when the patient is barefoot or wearing slippers.

3. **Hydration and Nutrition:**

- o Monitor and promote adequate hydration and nutrition to maintain skin elasticity and health, which is crucial for wound healing and overall foot condition.

Client Education for Elderly Foot Care

1. **Daily Foot Care Routine:**

    - o Educate patients and caregivers on the importance of daily foot inspections to catch potential problems early. Teach them what signs to look for, such as color changes, cuts, or unusual swelling.
    - o Instruct on the proper way to wash and thoroughly dry feet, especially between the toes, to prevent fungal infections.

2. **Proper Footwear:**

    - o Discuss the importance of wearing appropriate shoes that provide good support and fit well. Explain how ill-fitting shoes can lead to foot problems like bunions, corns, and ulcers.
    - o Advise on the selection of socks that do not restrict circulation.

3. **Exercise and Mobility:**

- Provide guidance on simple foot and ankle exercises that can be done safely at home to improve circulation and foot strength.
- Encourage participation in light, regular physical activities such as walking, swimming, or chair exercises tailored to their ability level.

4. **Professional Care and Follow-Up:**

    - Stress the importance of regular foot care appointments with healthcare professionals, especially for those with diabetes or poor circulation.
    - Encourage open communication about foot discomfort or pain during daily activities or routine care.

By integrating these nursing interventions, considerations, and educational strategies, healthcare providers can help elderly patients maintain healthy feet, prevent complications, and improve their overall quality of life.

Managing Arterial and Venous Diseases

Patients with arterial or venous diseases require special attention to prevent serious foot issues like ulcers or gangrene. Key considerations include:

Key Strategies:

- **Compression Therapy:** Using stockings to manage venous insufficiency.

- **Elevation:** Keeping feet elevated when resting to improve venous return.

- **Activity Modification:** Limiting activities that exacerbate symptoms.

Nursing Interventions for Managing Arterial and Venous Diseases

1. **Compression Therapy Management:**

   o Apply or supervise the application of prescribed compression stockings to ensure they fit properly and are used effectively to manage symptoms of venous insufficiency.

   o Monitor for signs of improper use or complications, such as skin irritation or worsening pain.

2. **Elevation and Positioning:**

   o Educate patients on the importance of elevating feet when resting to facilitate venous return and reduce swelling.

   o Assist patients in finding comfortable positions that promote blood flow without causing discomfort or pressure points.

3. **Activity Regulation and Exercise Promotion:**

   o Encourage regular, gentle exercise that promotes blood flow without overexerting the patient, such as swimming or walking, depending on individual tolerance.

- Advise on activity modifications to avoid prolonged standing or sitting, which can exacerbate symptoms.

Nursing Considerations for Arterial and Venous Diseases

1. **Risk Assessment and Monitoring:**

   - Regularly assess the patient's extremities for any signs of decreased perfusion such as coolness, pallor, or loss of hair, and venous symptoms like edema or varicose veins.
   - Closely monitor for early signs of complications, including ulcers or changes in skin coloration, which may indicate the onset of gangrene or severe infection.

2. **Care Coordination:**

   - Coordinate care with vascular specialists, wound care teams, and physical therapists to provide a multidisciplinary approach to managing the patient's condition.
   - Schedule regular follow-ups to adjust treatment plans based on the patient's progress and feedback.

3. **Patient Comfort and Pain Management:**

   - Address and manage pain through appropriate pharmacological and non-pharmacological methods.
   - Adjust compression therapy and elevation techniques to maximize comfort and effectiveness.

Client Education for Managing Arterial and Venous Diseases

1. **Understanding Disease Impact:**

   o Educate patients on how arterial and venous diseases affect their foot health and the risks associated with poor management.

   o Explain the mechanisms by which compression therapy and elevation help manage their condition.

2. **Proper Use of Compression Stockings:**

   o Instruct on how to correctly apply and remove compression stockings.

   o Discuss the importance of regular wear and care of stockings to maintain their therapeutic benefits.

3. **Lifestyle and Dietary Modifications:**

   o Advise on dietary changes that can improve blood flow and reduce venous pressure, such as reducing sodium intake to minimize swelling.

   o Recommend smoking cessation, as smoking can exacerbate arterial diseases.

4. **Recognizing and Responding to Complications:**

   o Teach patients to recognize the signs of potential complications, such as increased leg pain, changes in skin temperature or color, or the development of non-healing wounds.

> o Emphasize the importance of contacting healthcare providers immediately if these signs occur.

By integrating these interventions, considerations, and educational strategies, healthcare providers can effectively support patients with arterial and venous diseases, aiming to prevent serious complications and improve overall quality of life.

Preventive Strategies

Prevention of foot complications involves several overlapping strategies applicable to all special populations discussed:

- **Regular Monitoring:** Engaging with healthcare providers for frequent assessments.

- **Education:** Understanding the risks and symptoms of foot problems.

- **Community Support:** Leveraging support groups and resources for better foot care

Summary of Lessons Learned

- **Individualized Care:** Tailoring foot care approaches based on specific health conditions is crucial.

- **Prevention is Key:** Adopting preventive strategies significantly reduces the risk of severe complications.

- **Early Intervention:** Recognizing and addressing symptoms early can prevent adverse outcomes.

References

- American Diabetes Association. Guidelines for Diabetic Foot.

- National Institute on Aging. Elderly Footrace Recommendations.

- Vascular Health Clinics. Management of Venous Diseases: Best Practices.

This chapter emphasizes the importance of specialized foot care for diabetics, elderly patients, and individuals with arterial or venous diseases. By understanding and implementing tailored care strategies, complications can be significantly reduced, enhancing quality of life for these vulnerable populations.

Chapter 7: Orthotics and Prosthetics

Learning Objectives

By the end of this chapter, readers will be able to:

1. Describe the role and benefits of orthotics and prosthetic devices in foot care

2. Understand the process of fitting and adjusting orthotics and prosthetics.

3. Recognize the importance of patient education in the use of these devices.

4. Implement strategies to ensure optimal use and comfort of orthotics and prosthetics for patients.

Introduction

Orthotics and prosthetic devices play a critical role in enhancing mobility, reducing pain, and improving the quality of life for individuals with various foot-related issues. This chapter delves into the types, uses, and benefits of these devices, alongside detailed guidance on fitting, adjusting, and educating patients about their use.

Understanding Orthotics

Orthotics are custom-made or standard devices inserted into shoes to support, align, prevent, or correct deformities, or to improve the function of movable parts of the body.

Key Features and Benefits:

- **Support and Comfort:** Provides support to weak areas and reduces strain on the feet.

- **Correction of Foot Abnormalities:** Helps in aligning foot posture and correcting biomechanical foot issues.

- **Pain Relief:** Assists in distributing pressure evenly across the foot, reducing pain in sensitive areas.

Prosthetic Devices in Footrace

Prosthetics are artificial devices that replace missing parts of the body, often necessary after amputations due to diabetes, injury, or congenital conditions.

Key Features and Benefits:

- **Mobility Enhancement:** Enables individuals to regain mobility and functionality.

- **Improved Life Quality:** Offers a sense of normalcy and increases the capability to perform everyday activities.

- **Customization:** Tailored specifically to fit the needs and anatomy of each patient for optimal performance.

Fitting and Adjusting Orthotics and Prosthetics

Proper fitting and adjustment are paramount for the effectiveness of orthotics and prosthetics.

Best Practices:

- **Initial Assessment:** Detailed evaluation of the patient's foot anatomy and health condition.

- **Custom Design and Fitting:** Tailoring devices to meet individual needs and ensure comfort.
- **Follow-up Adjustments:** Regularly scheduled appointments to refine the fit as the patient adapts or as needs evolve.

Nursing Interventions for Orthotics and Prosthetics in Foot Care

1. **Assessment and Fitting:**
   - Assess the patient's foot anatomy and biomechanics to assist in the correct selection and fitting of orthotics or prosthetics. This includes measuring the foot, noting any deformities, and understanding the patient's daily activities and needs.
   - Work closely with orthotists or prosthetists to ensure the devices are properly fitted to avoid complications such as pressure sores or discomfort.

2. **Monitoring for Complications:**
   - Regularly inspect the skin, especially in areas where orthotics or prosthetics make contact. Look for signs of pressure ulcers, skin breakdown, or irritation.
   - Monitor the patient's gait and overall comfort while using orthotics or prosthetics, making adjustments as necessary to improve function and reduce discomfort.

3. **Care Coordination:**
   - Coordinate with a multidisciplinary team that may include podiatrists, physiotherapists, and

occupational therapists to provide comprehensive care tailored to the patient's specific needs.

- Ensure follow-up appointments are scheduled for ongoing assessment and adjustment of the orthotic or prosthetic devices.

Nursing Considerations for Orthotics and Prosthetics in Foot Care

1. **Patient Education and Training:**

    - Educate patients on the importance of wearing their orthotics or prosthetics as prescribed to prevent foot complications.
    - Instruct patients on how to properly care for and maintain their devices, including daily cleaning and inspection for damage.

2. **Lifestyle Adjustments:**

    - Discuss lifestyle and activity modifications with patients to enhance the effectiveness of their orthotic or prosthetic devices. This might include changes in types of physical activities or adjustments in daily routines.
    - Advise on the importance of gradual adaptation to the devices, allowing the body time to adjust to changes in biomechanics and pressure distribution.

3. **Comfort and Compliance:**

    - Address any comfort issues that may affect compliance. This includes ensuring the devices do not cause undue pain or discomfort, which can lead to non-use.

- Regularly assess and address any psychological impacts, such as frustration or self-consciousness related to device use.

Client Education for Orthotics and Prosthetics in Foot Care

1. **Proper Use and Maintenance:**

    - Teach patients how to properly put on and remove orthotics or prosthetics to minimize risk of injury.
    - Instruct on the regular maintenance of the devices, including how to check for wear and when to report potential problems.

2. **Recognizing Problems:**

    - Educate patients on the signs of potential problems related to orthotics and prosthetics, such as increased pain, new pressure areas, or changes in mobility.
    - Stress the importance of contacting their healthcare provider if they notice any of these signs or if they experience significant discomfort.

3. **Benefits of Proper Usage:**

    - Discuss the benefits of consistent and correct use of orthotics and prosthetics, emphasizing how these devices aid in mobility, reduce pain, and prevent further complications.
    - Encourage ongoing communication about their experiences with the devices to continuously optimize fit and function.

By integrating these interventions, considerations, and educational strategies, nurses can ensure that patients who require orthotics and prosthetics receive the necessary support to enhance their foot health and overall quality of life.

Education Strategies:

- **Proper Usage:** Instructing on how to wear and remove the devices correctly.

- **Maintenance Tips:** Providing guidelines on cleaning and caring for the devices.

- **Activity Recommendations:** Advising on suitable activities and any limitations.

Summary of Lessons Learned

- **Tailored Solutions:** Customization of orthotics and prosthetics is crucial for maximizing their benefits.

- **Continuous Care:** Regular follow-ups are essential for maintaining optimal fit and functionality.

- **Educational Empowerment:** Patient education enhances compliance and satisfaction with these devices.

References

- International Society for Prosthetics and Orthotics. Standards for Orthotic and Prosthetic Services.

- Podiatric Health Association. Guidelines on the Use of Orthotics in Clinical Practice.

This chapter provides a comprehensive overview of the critical role of orthotics and prosthetics in foot care, emphasizing the importance of proper fitting, adjustment, and patient education. These elements are crucial for maximizing the therapeutic benefits of these devices, ultimately leading to improved patient outcomes and quality of life.

Chapter 8: Pharmacological Treatments

Learning Objectives

By the end of this chapter, readers will be able to:

1. Identify common medications used in foot care and understand their indications.

2. Manage and mitigate the side effects associated with foot care medications.

3. Employ strategies to ensure patient compliance with pharmacological treatments.

Introduction

Pharmacological treatments play a vital role in managing various foot conditions, including infections, inflammation, and pain. This chapter explores the common medications used in foot care, their indications, side effects, and effective strategies to ensure patient compliance.

Common Medications and Their Indications

Medications in foot care are primarily used to treat infections, control pain, and reduce inflammation. Key classes of medications include:

Antibiotics

Used for treating bacterial infections, commonly prescribed antibiotics include:

- **Penicillins:** For soft tissue infections.

- **Cephalosporins:** For more severe or resistant infections.

Antifungals

Targeting fungal infections such as athlete's foot, common antifungals include:

- **Topical azoles** (e.g., clotrimazole)

- **Oral antifungals** (e.g., terbinafine)

Pain Relievers

For managing pain associated with foot conditions, medications include:

- **NSAIDs** (e.g., ibuprofen, naproxen): Reduce inflammation and alleviate pain.

- **Acetaminophen:** Used for pain relief without the anti-inflammatory effects.

Corticosteroids

Used to treat severe inflammation, corticosteroids can be administered topically or through injections at the site of discomfort.

Managing Side Effects

Each class of medication comes with potential side effects. Strategies for managing these include:

Monitoring

- **Routine Check-ups:** Monitoring patients for adverse reactions during treatment.
- **Blood Tests:** Ensuring no systemic effects are occurring, particularly with long-term antibiotic or corticosteroid use.

Medications That May Affect Foot Health

1. **Corticosteroids:**

   - **Impact:** Long-term use of corticosteroids can lead to skin thinning and decreased healing capacity, increasing the risk of foot ulcers.
   - **Conditions Affected:** Diabetic foot ulcers, other non-healing wounds.

2. **Vasodilators and Antihypertensives:**

   - **Impact:** These can cause swelling in the feet and ankles, complicating the assessment of edema due to underlying diseases.
   - **Conditions Affected:** Peripheral edema, venous insufficiency.

3. **Diuretics:**

   - **Impact:** While used to reduce edema, they can also lead to dehydration and decreased blood volume, potentially exacerbating peripheral neuropathy and other circulatory issues.
   - **Conditions Affected:** Diabetic neuropathy, peripheral arterial disease.

4. **Anticoagulants:**

- **Impact:** Increase the risk of bleeding, significant in the case of injuries or surgeries related to foot care. Can also lead to hematomas in the foot.
- **Conditions Affected:** Post-surgical bleeding, bruising.

5. **Beta-blockers:**
   - **Impact:** Can mask symptoms of worsening peripheral artery disease, such as leg pain and discomfort, which could prevent early detection and management.
   - **Conditions Affected:** Peripheral artery disease, claudication.

6. **Chemotherapy Drugs:**
   - **Impact:** Certain chemotherapeutic agents can cause peripheral neuropathy, leading to numbness, pain, or tingling in the feet, affecting balance and sensation.
   - **Conditions Affected:** Chemotherapy-induced peripheral neuropathy.

Nursing Considerations in Pharmacology and Foot Care

1. **Medication History and Monitoring:**
   - Regularly review the patient's medication list for any drugs that may impact foot health. This includes not only prescription drugs but also over-the-counter medications and supplements.
   - Monitor for signs of medication-induced complications, such as increased swelling, changes in skin integrity, or alterations in sensation.

2. **Patient Education:**

    o   Educate patients about the potential side effects of their medications on foot health. Ensure they understand the importance of reporting any new or worsening symptoms.

    o   Instruct patients on proper foot care practices, emphasizing the need for regular inspections and care routines to mitigate risks associated with their medications.

3. **Collaborative Care:**

    o   Collaborate with the healthcare team, including pharmacists and physicians, to manage or adjust medications that adversely affect foot health.

    o   Ensure that any changes in medication are closely monitored for effect on foot conditions.

4. **Holistic Assessment:**

    o   Conduct comprehensive assessments that consider the impact of medications on overall foot health. This includes evaluating vascular status, skin condition, and neurological status.

    o   Adjust foot care plans based on the patient's current medications and potential risks identified during assessments.

By understanding the pharmacological impacts on foot health and implementing thoughtful nursing considerations, nurses can significantly enhance care quality and prevent complications in patients with vulnerable foot conditions.

Ensuring Patient Compliance

Patient compliance is critical to the success of pharmacological treatments. Effective strategies include:

Clear Communication

- **Instructions:** Providing clear, understandable instructions for medication use.
- **Rationale:** Explaining the importance and expected outcomes of the medication regimen.

Follow-Up and Support

- **Regular Follow-Ups:** Scheduling appointments to assess treatment progress and adjust prescriptions as necessary.
- **Support Systems:** Establishing a support system to help patients manage their treatment schedules, especially for complex regimens.

Summary of Lessons Learned

- **Appropriate Medication Use:** Understanding the specific applications and limitations of each medication class is crucial for effective treatment.
- **Side Effect Management:** Proactively managing side effects can significantly improve patient comfort and treatment outcomes.

- **Enhancing Compliance:** Strategies that prioritize clear communication and patient education are essential for ensuring compliance and optimizing therapeutic effects.

References

- American Podiatric Medical Association.Pharmacological Approaches in Footrace

- Clinical Pharmacology of Footrace Comprehensive Guide to Drugs and Their Effects.

This chapter emphasizes the importance of pharmacological treatments in managing foot conditions, highlighting the need for careful medication selection, side effect management, and strategies to enhance patient compliance. Through proper understanding and application of these principles, healthcare providers can significantly improve patient outcomes in foot care

Chapter 9: Surgical Interventions

Learning Objectives

By the end of this chapter, readers will be able to:

1. Understand the range of surgical options available for both chronic and acute foot problems.

2. Identify the key considerations and preparations required for pre-operative care.

3. Manage post-operative care to enhance recovery and minimize complications.

4. Communicate effectively with patients about the expectations and potential risks of foot surgeries.

Introduction

Surgical interventions are often considered when conservative treatments fail to resolve foot problems or when rapid action is needed due to acute conditions. This chapter provides an overview of common surgical procedures for the foot, along with essential pre-operative and post-operative care guidelines.

Overview of Surgical Options

Surgical treatments can vary widely based on the specific foot issues being addressed. Common surgeries include:

Bunionectomy

For correcting deformities of the big toe caused by bunions.

Plantar Fascia Release

To relieve chronic heel pain associated with plantar fasciitis.

Metatarsal Surgery

For addressing issues related to the metatarsal bones, such as fractures or deformities.

Reconstructive Surgery

Used for severe deformities from conditions like flat feet or high arches.

Amputations

As a last resort, typically due to severe infections or circulatory problems.

Pre-Operative Care

Proper pre-operative preparation is crucial to the success of foot surgeries.

Key Preparations Include:

- **Medical Evaluation:** Assessing the patient's overall health to ensure readiness for surgery.
- **Medication Review:** Adjusting or halting medications that could complicate surgery, such as blood thinners.
- **Patient Education:** Discussing the procedure, potential risks, and expected outcomes to prepare the patient mentally and physically.

Post-Operative Care

Effective post-operative care is essential to ensure a smooth recovery and to prevent complications.

Key Aspects of Care:

- **Pain Management:** Using medications and techniques to manage post-surgical pain.

- **Wound Care:** Keeping surgical sites clean and monitored for signs of infection.

- **Physical Therapy:** Starting rehabilitation to restore function and mobility.

- **Follow-Up Visits:** Regular check-ups to monitor healing and address any concerns.

Summary of Lessons Learned

- **Surgical Precision:** Choosing the right surgical intervention based on specific patient conditions is critical.

- **Pre-Operative Planning:** Thorough preparation can significantly impact the surgical outcome.

- **Attentive Post-Operative Care:** Rigorous post-operative management is vital for successful recovery and patient satisfaction.

References

- American College of Foot and Ankle Surgeons. Guidelines for Foot and Ankle Surgery.

- Surgical Techniques in Podiatry. A Comprehensive Surgical Guide.

This chapter highlights the critical role of surgical interventions in treating both chronic and acute foot problems. Through detailed preparation and careful post-operative care, surgical outcomes can be optimized, enhancing both the functional and psychological well-being of patients.

Chapter 10: Preventive Care and Patient Education

Learning Objectives

By the end of this chapter, readers will be able to:

1. Understand the importance of preventive care in maintaining foot health.

2. Employ effective strategies to educate patients about foot health maintenance.

3. Develop and implement comprehensive care plans tailored to individual patient needs.

4. Recognize the role of continuous education in improving long-term patient outcomes.

Introduction

Preventive care and patient education are fundamental to maintaining foot health and preventing complications. This chapter explores effective strategies for educating patients and developing personalized care plans that emphasize preventive measures.

Importance of Preventive Care

Preventive care in podiatry aims to prevent the onset of foot problems before they develop into more serious conditions. It involves regular assessments, the use of appropriate footwear, and lifestyle modifications to enhance foot health.

Key Preventive Measures:

- **Regular Foot Examinations:** Encouraging annual or bi-annual checks to identify issues early.

- **Proper Footwear:** Educating about the importance of selecting shoes that offer proper support and fit.

- **Foot Hygiene:** Promoting daily routines that maintain foot cleanliness and health.

Strategies for Patient Education

Educating patients is crucial for effective preventive care. Strategies to enhance patient knowledge and engagement include:

Educational Materials

Providing brochures, videos, and online resources that patients can access at home to learn about foot care essentials.

Interactive Sessions

Conducting workshops and seminars where patients can actively learn about foot care and ask questions about their specific concerns.

Personalized Discussions

Tailoring discussions based on individual patient histories and risk factors, ensuring that each patient understands their unique needs and how to manage them.

Developing Comprehensive Care Plans

A comprehensive care plan addresses all aspects of a patient's foot health, tailored to their specific needs and lifestyle.

Components of a Comprehensive Care Plan:

- **Assessment:** Detailed evaluation of the patient's current foot health and risk factors.

- **Goal Setting:** Establishing clear, achievable goals related to improving or maintaining foot health.

- **Intervention Strategies:** Outlining specific actions, such as choosing appropriate footwear, implementing daily foot care routines, and scheduling regular follow-ups.

Implementation and Follow-Up

Ensuring that the care plan is followed through regular check-ins and adapting the plan as necessary to meet evolving needs.

Summary of Lessons Learned

- **Proactive Engagement:** Active patient participation is essential for the success of preventive care.

- **Customized Education:** Tailoring education and care plans to individual patient needs enhances understanding and engagement.

- **Ongoing Support:** Continuous support and follow-up are crucial to sustain positive outcomes in foot health.

References

- National Institute of Health Education. Guidelines for Patient Education in Podiatry.

- Comprehensive Preventive Care in Podiatry. Best Practices for Clinicians.

This chapter underscores the vital role of preventive care and patient education in podiatry, highlighting how these efforts can significantly reduce the incidence and severity of foot-related issues. Through thoughtful education and well-structured care plans, clinicians can empower patients to take an active role in maintaining their foot health, ultimately leading to better overall outcomes.

Chapter 11: Advancements in Footrace Nursing

Learning Objectives

By the end of this chapter, readers will be able to:

1. Identify the latest research and technologies in foot care

2. Understand current trends impacting the field of foot care nursing.

3. Anticipate future directions in therapy and patient management.

4. Integrate new findings and technologies into clinical practice for enhanced patient care.

Introduction

Footrace nursing is a dynamic field, continuously evolving as new research, technologies, and methodologies emerge. This chapter explores the latest advancements, highlighting how these innovations are shaping the future of therapy and patient management in foot care

Latest Research and Technologies

Recent years have seen significant breakthroughs in both the understanding and treatment of foot conditions. Key areas of advancement include:

Genetic Research

New insights into the genetic factors that contribute to foot and ankle disorders, paving the way for personalized medicine approaches.

Wound Healing Technologies

Innovations like smart bandages that track healing progress and deliver targeted treatments directly to the wound site.

Diagnostic Tools

Enhanced imaging technologies, such as high-resolution ultrasound, provide clearer, more detailed views of foot and ankle anatomy, improving diagnostic accuracy.

Current Trends in Footrace Nursing

The practice of foot care nursing is influenced by several prevailing trends:

Telemedicine

Remote consultations and follow-ups are becoming more prevalent, offering patients convenience and expanded access to specialized care.

Multidisciplinary Approaches

Collaboration across specialties, including podiatrists, physiotherapists, and diabetic specialists, to provide comprehensive care.

Patient-Centered Care

Increasing emphasis on tailoring treatment plans to individual patient preferences, lifestyles, and outcomes.

Future Directions in Therapy and Patient Management

Looking ahead, foot care nursing is set to be transformed by several emerging trends:

Regenerative Medicine

The use of stem cells and biologics to promote the regeneration of damaged tissues in the foot and ankle.

Robotics and Automation

Robot-assisted surgeries that provide greater precision and shorter recovery times are on the rise.

Predictive Analytics

Utilizing data analytics to predict patient outcomes and tailor interventions more precisely.

Summary of Lessons Learned

- **Embrace Innovation:** Staying current with technological and research advancements is crucial for improving patient care.

- **Holistic Approaches:** Effective treatment plans increasingly rely on interdisciplinary teams and holistic strategies.

- **Forward Thinking:** Anticipating and preparing for future changes in the field ensures that practitioners remain at the forefront of foot care nursing.

References

- International Journal of Footrace Nursing. (Year). Annual Review of Innovations in Footrace

- Future of Footrace Technology Conference. (Year). Proceedings and Keynote Speeches.

This chapter provides an in-depth look at the cutting-edge developments in foot care nursing, emphasizing the importance of integrating new research and technologies into everyday practice. By understanding and adopting these advancements, foot care professionals can enhance their approach to patient care and prepare for future shifts in the healthcare landscape.

Chapter 12: Building a Footrace Practice

Learning Objectives

By the end of this chapter, readers will be able to:

1. Identify the essential steps for setting up a successful foot care practice.

2. Understand key legal and business considerations in the healthcare sector.

3. Implement effective marketing strategies to attract and retain patients.

4. Develop a growth-oriented business plan that adapts to changes in the healthcare landscape.

Introduction

Building a successful foot care practice requires more than medical expertise; it also involves understanding the nuances of business, legal regulations, and marketing. This chapter outlines the foundational elements of establishing and managing a thriving foot care practice.

Setting Up a Footrace Practice

The initial setup of a foot care practice involves several critical steps:

Location and Facilities

Choosing a location that is accessible to your target patient demographic and setting up a facility that meets their needs in terms of comfort and equipment.

Licensing and Compliance

Ensuring all necessary medical licenses are obtained and that the practice complies with local healthcare regulations and standards.

Staffing

Hiring qualified staff, including additional foot care specialists, nurses, and administrative personnel, to provide the best patient care and support operational needs.

Legal Considerations

Navigating the legal landscape is crucial for any healthcare practice:

Patient Privacy and Data Security

Understanding and implementing measures to comply with patient privacy laws.

Professional Liability

Securing appropriate malpractice insurance to protect against potential legal claims.

Business Considerations

Running a foot care practice also involves key business operations:

Financial Management

Setting up efficient billing systems, managing costs, and ensuring profitability.

Strategic Planning

Developing a business plan that includes clear objectives, revenue targets, and strategies for growth and expansion.

Marketing Your Practice

Effective marketing is essential to attract and retain patients:

Branding

Creating a strong brand that communicates the values and specialties of your practice.

Digital Marketing

Utilizing online platforms like a professional website, social media, and local SEO to increase visibility.

Community Engagement

Participating in community events and health fairs to raise awareness and build local networks.

Summary of Lessons Learned

- **Comprehensive Preparation:** Thorough preparation in legal, business, and facility setup is essential for a successful launch.

- **Ongoing Development:** Continuously updating business and marketing strategies in response to market changes and patient feedback.

- **Community Focus:** Building strong community connections enhances patient trust and practice reputation.

References

- National Association of Podiatric Medical Practices. Guide to Starting a Podiatric Practice.

- Successful Footrace Practice Management. Insights and Strategies.

This chapter provides a roadmap for setting up and managing a successful foot care practice, emphasizing the importance of legal compliance, effective business operations, and proactive marketing. By understanding and implementing these elements, practitioners can establish a robust foundation for their practice and foster sustainable growth.

Chapter 13: Ethics and Professionalism in Footrace Nursing

Learning Objectives

By the end of this chapter, readers will be able to:

1. Identify common ethical dilemmas specific to foot care nursing.

2. Apply ethical principles to resolve conflicts and make informed decisions.

3. Maintain a high standard of professionalism and empathy in clinical practice.

4. Develop strategies to enhance patient trust and ethical care delivery.

Introduction

Ethics and professionalism are foundational to effective foot care nursing, guiding interactions with patients and shaping the delivery of care. This chapter explores the ethical dilemmas unique to foot care and discusses how to uphold professionalism and empathy in clinical settings.

Ethical Dilemmas in Footrace Nursing

Footrace nurses often face specific ethical challenges that require careful consideration and decision-making.

Patient Autonomy vs. Recommended Care

Balancing respect for patient autonomy with the need to recommend treatments that are in the patient's best interest can be challenging, especially when patients are reluctant to follow advice due to personal beliefs or financial constraints.

Confidentiality and Privacy

Maintaining patient confidentiality, especially in small community settings where personal and professional lives may intersect, poses unique challenges.

Resource Allocation

Deciding how to fairly allocate limited resources, such as time or specialized care equipment, among patients who need them.

Maintaining Professionalism and Empathy

Professionalism and empathy are critical in ensuring that ethical standards are met while providing patient-centered care.

Developing Empathy

Fostering an empathetic understanding of each patient's situation, which enhances trust and communication.

Upholding Standards

Consistently adhering to clinical guidelines and professional codes of conduct, even in challenging situations.

Communication Skills

Enhancing communication skills to clearly and compassionately convey treatment options and expectations to patients.

Strategies for Ethical Decision-Making

Implementing frameworks for ethical decision-making can help nurses address dilemmas effectively.

Ethical Frameworks

Using established ethical frameworks to guide decisions, such as the four basic principles of medical ethics: autonomy, beneficence, non-maleficence, and justice.

Team Consultations

Engaging with a multidisciplinary team to gather diverse perspectives and reach consensus on ethical issues.

Continuing Education

Participating in ongoing ethics training and professional development to stay informed about emerging ethical issues and best practices.

Summary of Lessons Learned

- **Ethical Awareness:** Recognizing and understanding the ethical dilemmas specific to foot care is essential for responsible practice.

- **Empathetic Practice:** Maintaining empathy and professionalism enhances patient relationships and care outcomes.

- **Dynamic Solutions:** Ethical practice requires continuous learning and adaptation to new challenges and scenarios.

References

- Ethics in Podiatric Medicine. National Council on Podiatric Medical Ethics.

- Professional Conduct in Footrace Nursing. Guidelines and Case Studies.

This chapter underscores the importance of ethics and professionalism in foot care nursing, providing insights into navigating complex ethical dilemmas and maintaining high standards of care. By cultivating a deep understanding of these principles, foot care nurses can build stronger, more trusting relationships with their patients and uphold the integrity of their profession.

Chapter 14: Conclusion: The Future of Footrace Nursing

Learning Objectives

By the end of this chapter, readers will be able to:

1. Reflect on the evolving role of foot care nurses in the healthcare system.//
2. Recognize the importance of continuous education and specialization in advancing foot care nursing.
3. Understand the impact of technological advancements on the practice of foot care nursing.
4. Anticipate future challenges and opportunities in the field of foot care nursing.

Introduction

The role of foot care nurses has dramatically evolved and will continue to do so amidst rapidly advancing medical technologies and changing healthcare landscapes. This concluding chapter reflects on these transformations and underscores the importance of ongoing education and specialization.

The Evolving Role of Footrace Nurses

Footrace nurses are increasingly recognized as vital in preventative health, chronic disease management, and specialized patient care. Their role has expanded from basic care provision to include roles such as:

Specialist Practitioners

Becoming experts in managing complex foot health issues, such as diabetic foot care and wound management.

Educators

Providing patient education and advocating for foot health as an integral part of overall well-being.

Researchers

Engaging in research activities to advance the science of foot care and improve care protocols.

The Importance of Continuous Education

As the field of foot care nursing evolves, continuous professional development becomes essential.

Specialization

Pursuing specialization in areas like diabetic care, pediatric foot care, or sports injuries can enhance career opportunities and patient outcomes.

Lifelong Learning

Engaging in ongoing learning through workshops, seminars, and advanced degrees to stay updated with the latest practices and technologies.

Impact of Technological Advancements

Technological innovations are set to further revolutionize the practice of foot care nursing.

Telemedicine

Expanding the reach of foot care nurses to remote or underserved populations through virtual consultations and care management.

Advanced Diagnostics

Utilizing state-of-the-art imaging and diagnostic tools to provide more accurate assessments and personalized treatment plans.

Future Challenges and Opportunities

The future of foot care nursing will be shaped by several key factors:

Demographic Shifts

Addressing the needs of an aging population and the associated increase in chronic foot health issues.

Policy and Regulation

Navigating changes in healthcare policies and regulations that impact practice scopes and patient care delivery.

Global Health Trends

Responding to global health trends, including the rise in chronic diseases and the need for more holistic, multidisciplinary approaches to healthcare.

Summary of Lessons Learned

- **Adaptive Role:** Footrace nurses must continue to adapt to new roles and responsibilities in response to evolving healthcare needs.

- **Emphasis on Education:** Ongoing education and specialization are critical for keeping pace with advancements in the field.

- **Technological Integration:** Embracing new technologies will be crucial for improving patient care and expanding practice capabilities.

References

- Future Trends in Podiatric Nursing. Global Insights.

- Continuous Professional Development in Nursing. Guidelines and Best Practices.

This chapter provides a comprehensive overview of the current state and future prospects of foot care nursing, emphasizing the need for adaptability, continuous learning, and specialization. As foot care nurses embrace these elements, they will not only enhance their professional development but also significantly contribute to the advancement of the field and the well-being of their patients.

Chapter 15: Breakdown of a Footrace Nursing Session

Learning Objectives

By the end of this chapter, readers will be able to:

1. Identify the essential tools and supplies needed for a foot care nursing session.

2. Understand the step-by-step process of a typical foot care nursing session.

3. Utilize proper charting techniques and terminology relevant to foot care

4. Apply effective foot care techniques to enhance patient outcomes.

Introduction

A well-organized foot care nursing session is critical for effective patient care. This chapter provides a detailed breakdown of the session, including the necessary tools and supplies, a step-by-step guide to the procedure, and best practices in charting and foot care techniques.

Tools and Supplies Needed for Footrace Nursing

Before beginning a session, ensure that all necessary tools and supplies are available and in good condition. Essential items include:

- **Nail Clippers, Nippers and Files:** For trimming and shaping nails.

- **Scalpels and Scissors:** For removing dead skin and calluses.
- **Antiseptics:** For cleaning the feet and preventing infections.
- **Moisturizers:** To keep the skin hydrated.
- **Gloves and Masks:** For hygiene and infection control.
- **Foot Basins and Towels:** For washing and drying feet.
- **Diagnostic Tools:** Such as monofilaments for diabetic neuropathy testing.

Step-by-Step Breakdown of a Footrace Nursing Session

A typical foot care session involves several key steps:

1. Preparation

- **Sanitize Tools:** Ensure all tools are sterilized.
- **Set Up the Work Area:** Arrange all supplies for easy access.

2. Initial Assessment

- **Patient Consultation:** Discuss any foot problems or concerns.
- **Visual and Physical Examination:** Check for any abnormalities or signs of infection.

3. Foot Washing

- **Soak Feet:** Use warm water and mild soap.
- **Dry Thoroughly:** Especially between the toes.

4. Nail Care

- **Trimming:** Cut nails straight across to prevent ingrown toenails.
- **Filing:** Smooth edges to avoid sharpness.

5. Callus and Corn Management

- **Identify Areas:** Locate calluses and corns.
- **Gentle Removal:** Use appropriate tools, taking care not to cause injury.

6. Moisturizing and Massage

- **Apply Moisturizer:** To prevent dryness.
- **Foot Massage:** To improve circulation.

7. Final Assessment and Advice

- **Review the Feet:** Ensure all issues are addressed.
- **Provide Care Recommendations:** Advise on daily foot care routines.

Charting and Terminology

Accurate charting and the use of proper terminology are vital for effective communication and documentation.

Key Components of Charting:

- **Patient Information:** Name, date, and medical history.
- **Observations:** Detailed notes on findings from the foot examination.
- **Actions Taken:** Treatments applied during the session.
- **Patient Instructions:** Care instructions given to the patient.
- **Follow-Up Notes:** Recommendations for future sessions.

Techniques in Footrace

Effective foot care techniques are essential for patient comfort and health.

- **Gentle Handling:** Always handle feet gently to avoid discomfort.
- **Hygienic Practices:** Maintain strict hygiene to prevent infections.
- **Patient Education:** Teach patients how to care for their feet at home.

Summary of Lessons Learned

- **Preparation Is Key:** Proper preparation ensures a smooth and effective session.
- **Thoroughness and Attention to Detail:** Meticulous care can prevent many foot problems.

- **Effective Communication:** Clear communication and professional documentation are crucial for ongoing foot care management.

References

- Comprehensive Footrace in Nursing. Protocol and Best Practices.
- Tools and Techniques for Effective Footrace A Practical Guide.

This chapter offers a comprehensive overview of conducting a foot care nursing session, from preparation through follow-up. By mastering these steps, tools, and techniques, foot care nurses can provide exceptional care that significantly improves their patients' foot health and overall well-being.

Sample of a Basic Chart Form

Footrace Nursing Documentation Form

Patient Information:

- **Name:** _____
- **Date of Birth:** _____
- **Patient ID:** _____
- **Date of Visit:** _____
- **Referring Physician:** _____

Medical History:

- **Diabetes:** Yes / No
- **Peripheral Neuropathy:** Yes / No
- **Arterial Disease:** Yes / No
- **Venous Insufficiency:** Yes / No
- **Other Relevant Conditions:**
  _____

Current Medications:
_____

Allergies (medications/environmental):
_____

Initial Assessment:

- **Reason for Visit:**
  _____

- **Patient's Main Concerns:**
  _____

- **Visual Inspection:**

    o **Skin Condition:** Normal / Dry / Cracked / Other

    o **Nail Condition:** Normal / Thickened / Fungal / Other

    o **Presence of Calluses/Corns:** Yes / No

    o **Presence of Wounds/Ulcers:** Yes / No

- **Physical Examination:**

    o **Pulses:** Present / Absent (Dorsalis Pedis, Posterior Tibial)

    o **Sensation Test Results:** Normal / Decreased / Absent

    o **Foot Structure:** Normal / Flat Feet / High Arches / Other

    o **Mobility Issues:** None / Mild / Moderate / Severe

Procedure Performed:

- **Foot Washing:** Done / Not Required

- **Nail Care:** Trimmed / Filed / Not Required

- **Callus/Corn Management:** Removed / Reduced / Not Required

- **Skin Care:** Moisturizing / Treatment Applied / Not Required
- **Massage:** Performed / Not Required

Observations:

- **Findings:**
  _____
  ___

- **Complications During Session:** None / Minor / Major
  - **Details:**
    _____
    ___

Plan and Recommendations:

- **Follow-Up Care:**
  _____

- **Home Care Instructions:**
  _____

- **Next Appointment Scheduled:** Yes / No
  - **Date:** _____

Nurse's Notes:

- **Comments:**
  _____

- **Nurse Name:**
  _____

- **Signature:**
  _____

- **Date:**
  _____

Tips and Tricks for Effective Footrace Nursing

As a foot care nurse, you have the critical task of not only treating but also preventing foot-related issues in your patients. Below are some essential tips and tricks that can help you enhance the effectiveness of your foot care practice, ensuring better patient outcomes and increased satisfaction.

1. Prioritize Patient Education

Educating patients is one of the most crucial aspects of foot care Spend time teaching your patients about proper foot hygiene, the importance of wearing suitable footwear, and the correct way to trim their nails. Use diagrams, models, or digital content to help them understand their conditions and the care procedures they should follow at home.

2. Stay Updated with the Latest Techniques

Footrace is an evolving field, with new treatments and technologies constantly emerging. Regularly participate in workshops, seminars, and continuing education courses to stay current with the latest advancements in foot care This ongoing learning will enable you to provide the most effective treatments to your patients.

3. Use High-Quality Tools

The quality of the tools you use can significantly affect the outcome of your care. Invest in high-quality, durable instruments such as nail clippers, files, and skin care tools that are specifically designed for professional use in foot care Regularly sterilize and maintain your tools to prevent infections and ensure they perform as needed.

4. Develop a Systematic Assessment Process

Create a structured approach to assessing patient feet, which should include checking for any abnormalities such as cuts, blisters, calluses, and signs of infection. A systematic assessment ensures you don't miss any issues and provides a thorough record for tracking changes over time.

5. Implement Tailored Care Plans

Recognize that each patient is unique and tailor your care plans accordingly. Consider factors like age, mobility, underlying health conditions (e.g., diabetes, vascular disease), and lifestyle when creating care plans. Customized care plans not only address the specific needs of each patient but also improve compliance and effectiveness of treatments.

6. Focus on Preventive Care

Prevention is key in foot care nursing. Encourage regular check-ups and intervene early when potential issues are identified. Teach patients preventive measures such as wearing the right kind of socks, using appropriate moisturizers, and conducting daily foot inspections.

7. Build Rapport and Trust

A good nurse-patient relationship is based on trust and communication. Take the time to listen to your patients' concerns and experiences. Empathetic listening can significantly impact patient comfort and willingness to comply with treatment protocols.

8. Optimize Your Workspace

Ensure your workspace is ergonomically set up to prevent strain on your body, especially given the nature of foot care nursing, which often requires prolonged periods of sitting or bending. An optimized workspace can improve your efficiency and reduce fatigue.

9. Maintain Patient Privacy and Dignity

Always respect patient privacy and dignity, especially during potentially uncomfortable treatments. Use appropriate draping techniques and ensure the patient feels secure and respected throughout their care session.

10. Document Thoroughly

Accurate and detailed documentation is crucial. Record every session's findings and treatments, along with any patient-reported symptoms and outcomes. Good records help monitor progress over time and are essential for legal compliance and quality assurance.

11. Consider Supplies: Disposable vs. Reusable

Decide whether to use disposable or reusable tools. Reusable tools require strict sanitization between uses, with an autoclave being the gold standard for sterilization. Also, consider the costs and financing of such equipment, which can be a significant investment but essential for maintaining high standards of care.

12. Setting Price and Upselling

Consider your costs carefully. The average foot care session will take between 45 minutes to an hour. Upselling products like creams, compression socks, or specialty treatments can significantly boost your income. Additionally, offering to do hand nail care for a small extra fee is a great way to capitalize on the income potential of each visit.

13. Business Generation

Actively seek out opportunities to generate business. Contact your local chamber of commerce and local churches to set up clinics. Approach local retirement homes, long-term care homes, and adult lifestyle communities to offer your services. Make use of internet technologies and social media to promote your services and connect with potential clients.

By incorporating these tips and tricks into your practice, you can elevate the level of care you provide and ensure your patients receive the best possible outcomes. Remember, effective foot care nursing not only addresses current problems but also prevents future issues, enhancing overall health and mobility for your patients.

Author Bio:

Chad Peterson is a registered practical nurse based in Ontario, Canada, with a rich background in both nursing and medical laboratory sciences. After completing his nursing studies at Sir Sanford Fleming College, Chad specialized in diabetic foot care, earning a certification from Ruth Rutan Footrace His academic pursuits also include a diploma in Medical Laboratory Technician from Medix College, complemented by provincial licenses in nursing and medical laboratory technology through the College of Nurses Ontario and the Ontario Society of Medical Technicians (OSMT), respectively.

Chad is committed to continuous professional development, having participated in advanced training programs in dialysis, palliative care, and wound care management. His diverse professional experience spans roles as a personal support worker in long-term care and community settings, and as a medical laboratory technician in clinical research and community environments. Currently, Chad practices nursing in hospital, long-term care, and community settings where he employs an evidence-based, holistic, and client-centered approach to care.

In his debut book on nursing foot care, Chad combines his extensive clinical expertise with a practical approach, aiming to empower nurses and healthcare professionals with the knowledge and skills necessary to provide exceptional foot care His book is an essential resource for those committed to enhancing patient outcomes through specialized foot care

Link to my Linkedin Profile
https://www.linkedin.com/in/chadpeterson2/